Be a Cancer Thriver

POEMS AND SCRIPTURES TO HELP YOU ON YOUR JOURNEY

JANIS COX

Butterfly Beacons

Published by Butterfly Beacons www.janiscox.cox
Library and Archives Canada Cataloguing in Publication

Cox, Janis, 1949

Be a Cancer Thriver/Janis Cox

ISBN 978-1-990870-01-9 (print)

1. Title

Contents

Introduction

How to explain the feelings and the emotions of those first months with cancer? I looked at my journals because it's hard trying to remember back then. I've moved forward and thought I would share some of what happened during that time with journal entries and my poetry.

My first knowledge that something might be wrong came with a phone call (September 2, 2021) for a recall after a routine mammogram (six days before). They wanted to take the mammogram again? Since the age of 50, I had a mammogram. Every time I received a letter saying everything is okay,

This time, I was stunned. I didn't believe it. It must be a technical error, I told myself. I learned from friends that recalls normally come back negative. That helped assured me all was okay. The recall was for September 14. I kept reading the Bible, praying and trying to stay calm. By always counting God's blessings every day, I kept focused on the present. A positive attitude always helps. If I found myself going down the "what if" trail, I would immediately pray for calmness. My daily walks helped me, too. They scheduled the recall mammogram quickly.

Journal Entry September 5

I've been calmer about mammogram recall—Your wraparound presence helps me. H.E.L.P. (Having Everything Lifted in Prayer) My recall will be on September 14. Sometimes I feel, Lord, that none of this is going on.

I had the mammogram and waited. I assumed it was nothing because really I was 72. Why would I get cancer now?

On September 16, the next phone call asked me to come back for a biopsy. Once again, I heard that 75% of these turn out to be negative.

Journal Entry September 17

Lots going on. I think I got some things done. I am trying to be an encouragement to others. All this writing I have done and now want to publish.

During this time, I have been working on *Growing Through God's Word* 2 (my second in the series—a set of devotionals).

I read Psalm 1 verse 3:

That person is like a tree planted by streams of water, which yields its fruit in season and whose leaf does not wither—whatever they do prospers. (NIV)

Looking at this scripture, I could see the analogy of being planted close to the water. I kept close to that water (Jesus) and He fed me and strengthened me.

Then it was biopsy time, September 24. Back to the same place as the mammograms. The procedure wasn't too bad. The technicians and the doctor were great. There was a problem with the position I had to stay in, as my neck, at that time, felt tight (that's all fixed now). I kept praying, and all went well.

Time to wait again.

For God did not give us a spirit of timidity or cowardice or fear, but [He has given us a spirit] of power and of love and of sound judgment and personal discipline [abilities that result in a calm, well-balanced mind and self-control]. (2 Timothy 1:7 AMP)

The morning of the day I received the diagnosis of cancer from my doctor, I read this:

Test me, O LORD, and try me, examine my heart and my mind. (Psalm 26:2, NIV)

Journal Entry October 1

Motives. What is behind me? Who is the real me? (I asked myself questions to find out how I really felt.)

Psalm 51:10

Create in me a pure heart, O God, and renew a steadfast spirit within me. (NIV)

In The Message it read, "order a battery of tests." Oh my, exactly what I have been going through.

Roman 8:1-11

This compares life through the flesh with life through the Spirit. Spirit desires life and peace. The Spirit lives within me.

1 Timothy 1:17

Now to the King eternal, immortal, invisible, the only God, be honor and glory for ever and ever. Amen. (NIV)

After reading and studying these scriptures, I was ready to face whatever God had in store for me.

6:30 pm on October 1, 2021, I got the call.

"I am so sorry, but you have cancer. I have called a specialist and she will be in touch with you next week."

Journal Entry October 2

This is not what I had hoped and prayed for. But I know You only have good planned through this. Your glory. Your testimony. May my children find You through this time. That is my heartfelt prayer.

I ended this morning's study session with Psalm 26:12. This Psalm has become the one I repeat if I feel myself swayed by worry.

My feet stand on level ground;
in the great congregation I will praise the Lord. (NIV)

My journalling hasn't ended. I continue to read God's Word each day. I encourage others to read with me. The trials will not end, but with God walking with us, we can take each trial one step at a time.

Poetry

I have always loved writing poetry. When I taught grade one, I made a poem or story each week on the topic we were studying. I would put these into their Bedtime Story Books. The children took them home to read for a week, to learn vocabulary and sentence structure. When they came back on Friday, we would read our story again together.

When I first committed to following Jesus, I wrote in a daily journal. I studied selected scriptures and asked God many questions. As I waited for the answer, it usually came in poetical form. During those first years, I wrote 150 poems (not yet in print).

Lately, I have enjoyed writing poetry in a new style: Abecedarian Poetry. This poetry uses the alphabet to start each verse. Psalm 119 is an abecedarian poem. I like the structure as it makes me think of the next word or phrase.

Have you tried writing poetry? It's a significant form of expression, especially after reading scripture.

Many of the poems in this book are abecedarian poems and the others are free style.

Thank You

I would like to thank the following people for help in giving me feedback for my book.

Carissa Jones
Kimberley Payne
Ida Adams
Julie Goodwin
Valerie Secor
Susan Elizabeth Henson
Nancy Booth
Linda Fode

Thank you for your time and commitment.

Blessings,

Janis

Wrap Around God

Psalm 7:10

God, your wraparound presence is my shield.
You bring victory to all who are pure in heart. (TPT)

I feel your presence
You sustain me
The word cancer
Is frightening
It makes everything

Stop

But then I realize
It makes everything

Go

I know You are leading me
To new discoveries
Opening my heart to love
Your love

Being still in Your arms
I can feel the beat of my heart
I can feel the breath in my lungs

You sustain me
You will give me strength
We are on this cancer journey
Together

October 3rd, 2021

Psalm 84:9-11

God, your wraparound presence is our defense.
In your kindness look upon the faces of your anointed ones. (TPT)

Psalm 62:2

He alone is my safe place;
his wraparound presence always protects me. (TPT)

Psalm 62:6

For he alone is my safe place.
His wraparound presence always protects me
as my champion defender.
There's no risk of failure with God!
So why would I let worry paralyze me,
even when troubles multiply around me? (TPT)

Psalm 16:8-11

I keep my eyes always on the Lord.
With him at my right hand, I will not be shaken.
Therefore my heart is glad and my tongue rejoices;
my body also will rest secure,
because you will not abandon me to the realm of the dead,
nor will you let your faithful one see decay.
You make known to me the path of life;
you will fill me with joy in your presence,
with eternal pleasures at your right hand. (NIV)

May I pray for you and me?

Heavenly Father, sustainer of all life, come close to us at this time. We feel perplexed, scared and weary. Help us rely more on You for strength and peace. In Jesus' Name. Amen.

Journal Your Thoughts

But Here I Stand

Psalm 26:12

My feet stand on level ground
In the great assembly I will praise the LORD. (ESV)

As I stand firm
In God's truth
The world may sway
But here I stand

I wait
For my next step
The goal He sets before me
Is to excite others
To read His Word

Nothing can knock me over
Not even a cancer diagnosis
Because I have Jesus
Surrounding me.

October 4, 2021

Whoever walks in integrity walks securely,
but whoever takes crooked paths will be found out. (Proverbs 10:9, NIV)

May I pray for you and me?

Lord, we are hanging on to You. No matter what is going on around us, we focus on Your goodness and mercy. We will not be shaken. In Jesus' Name. Amen.

Journal Your Thoughts

Walk With God

Psalm 55:2

Hear me and answer me.
My thoughts trouble me and I am distraught. (NIV)

Troubled thoughts on hearing a cancer diagnosis.
Where do I go?
To God of course.

I am on a new adventure.

Another day
Between me and
Cancer

Death doesn't frighten me
Even though it's always there

Freedom in Jesus
God I seek
Heaven is real

Into new adventures
Jesus at my side
Keeps me calm
Loves continually
Makes me strong

Nothing will shake my faith
Opens new thoughts
Puts the world aside

Questions abound
Rest is essential
Safety in love

Teaching me to trust
Understanding His Word
Voice of God

Walk with Him
eXpecting
Your Presence, Lord, this is not the
Zed

October 5, 2021

But God has surely listened
and has heard my prayer. (Psalm 66:19, NIV)

May I pray for you and me?

Heavenly Father, we thank You for the gift of prayer. We thank You, too, for Your Word – the Word of truth. Help us understand it. Help us walk with You. In Jesus' Name. Amen.

Journal Your Thoughts

I Study

1 Timothy 5:21

Do nothing out of favoritism. (NIV)

I know Jesus
You are in charge

I look to You for strength
I look to You for comfort

As I sit after studying Your Word
The vastness of the Word
Astounds me
Understanding it would take more than a lifetime

Each day a new nugget appears:
"Do nothing out of favouritism."

I see this broken every day
The world is full of favouritism
You scratch my back
I'll scratch yours
Under the table deals

What happened to righteousness?

O, Lord, reveal evil practices
Open wide the cracks
Let truth pour out

You have the plan, Lord
What part do you want me to play?

I am listening
I will act.

October 6, 2021

A new command I give you: Love one another. As I have loved you, so you must love one another. (John 13:34, NIV)

May I pray for you and me?

Heavenly Father, Author of life, Redeemer. Help us to remember that we are all Your creation. We are equal to one another. Help us not to judge others. Help us learn to love our neighbours. In Jesus' Name. Amen.

Journal Your Thoughts

Faith in God

Journal Entry:

Faith is developed through use.

Prayer
Reading the Bible

Romans 15:13

May the God of hope fill you with all joy and peace as you trust in him, so that you may overflow with hope by the power of the Holy Spirit (NIV)

Any
Belief
Can
Die
Even
Faith in God

Hatred
Insists on
Justice (man's not God's)
Keeps
Love
Muted
Not allowing
Peace

Quietness and
Rest to
See the
Truth and
Unveil His
Voice
Which
eXpresses His
Yearning and
Zeal for me and you.

October 7, 2021

Rejoice always, pray continually, give thanks in all circumstances; for this is God's will for you in Christ Jesus. (1 Thessalonians 5:16-18, NIV)

May I pray for you and me?

Heavenly Father, help us to find the joy You give by resting in You. Help us remember to thank You each day. By the power of the Holy Spirit, bring peace into our hearts. In Jesus' Name. Amen

Journal Your Thoughts

Day by Day

Psalm 90:12

*Teach us to number our days,
that we may gain a heart of wisdom. (NIV)*

Another
Busy
Colourful
Day

Everything
Feels
Good

Hold
Intensely to
Jesus

Keep
Living
Mindfully

Nothing
Opens
Peace
Quite like
Rest

Seek
To
Understand
Volumes of His
Word

eXpect to find
Youthful
Zeal

October 10, 2021

And may your hearts be fully committed to the Lord our God, to live by his decrees and obey his commands, as at this time. (1 Kings 8:61, NIV)

May I pray for you and me?

Heavenly Father, we know we need to read Your Word. Help us to do this consistently. But also, help us to understand what we read. Keep our eyes focused on Jesus. In His Name we pray. Amen.

Journal Your Thoughts

Anno Domini

1 John 2:15

Don't set the affections of your heart on this world or in loving the things of the world. The love of the Father and the love of the world are incompatible. (TPT)

Before
Christ
Death then after Christ

Eternity
Freedom
Gate to
Heaven

In walks
Jesus
Keeper of
Love
Master of all

Notifies us
Of
Paradise
Questions
Reality
Shows us
Truth

Understand His
Visit
Who died on the
X
Yet broke the
Z

October 25, 2021

Beloved children, our love can't be an abstract theory we only talk about, but a way of life demonstrated through our loving deeds. (1 John 3:18, TPT)

May I pray for you and me?

Heavenly Father, thank You for Jesus. Help us be mindful of all that He did for us, the impact He has made on our lives. He has reconnected us with God and living with Him for all eternity. In Jesus' Name. Amen.

Journal Your Thoughts

As I Wait

Psalm 28:2

Hear my cry for mercy
as I call to you for help,
as I lift up my hands
toward your Most Holy Place.

As I wait
Before surgery I
Can feel
Deep down
Every prayer
From the faithful

God
Heals

In fact
Jesus
Keeps
Loving
Me

Nothing can
Obstruct those
Prayers

Quietness
Reflect while I
Sit here

Taking time
Understanding that those
Voices
Would
eXcite God

Your
Zeal, dear faithful ones

October 26, 2021

Therefore confess your sins to each other and pray for each other so that you may be healed. The prayer of a righteous person is powerful and effective. (James 5:16, NIV)

May I pray for you and me?

Heavenly Father, we thank You for giving us prayer partners, those who will pray with us and for us. Your Word speaks of the power of prayer. May we continue to pray as You taught us, Jesus. In Your Name, we pray. Amen.

Journal Your Thoughts

We Need God

Psalm 146:3

Do not put your trust in princes,
in human beings, who cannot save. (NIV)

Anger
Brings
Chaos

Don't let
External words and thoughts
Focus us on
Grasping
Hurt

Internal thoughts of
Jesus
Keep us full of
Love – and
Make Him
Near – it
Opens a place for
Peace
Quickens our
Responsive tie with His
Spirit

To
Ultimately
Voice
What God
eXpects

Your full desire for Him
Zealousness.

October 30, 2021

Trust instead in the one who lavishes upon us all good things, fulfilling our every need. (1 Timothy 6:17b, TPT)

Be alert and guard your heart from greed and from always wishing for what you don't have. (Luke 12:15, TPT)

May you be richly rewarded by the Lord, the God of Israel, under whose wings you have come to take refuge. (Ruth 2:12, NIV)

May I pray for you and me?

Heavenly Father, oh there is so much to learn. Help us to be alert to what You want and also what You don't want. Help us be in touch with the Holy Spirit as we work at getting to know You better. In Jesus' Name. Amen.

Journal Your Thoughts

Adopted

James 1:21

Therefore, get rid of all moral filth and the evil that is so prevalent, and humbly accept the word planted in you, which can save you. (NIV)

Adopted
Before time

Christ came with a
Determined
Effort to
Find us

God sent
Him
Intentionally

Jesus
Kept that promise to bring us
Life

Making connection possible
Never forsaking us

Opening communication through
Prayer – letting us
Question – teaching us

Righteousness – letting our
Spirits soar

Toppling world's
Understandings

Voicing
Who He is

eXpanding our
Youth till our
Zed

November 2, 2021

In simple humility, let our gardener, God, landscape you with the Word, making a salvation-garden of your life. (James 1:21, MSG)

May I pray for you and me?

Heavenly Father, guide us in our daily lives. Teach us to know who You are. Help us read Your Word and let it become a part of us. In Jesus' Name. Amen.

Journal Your Thoughts

Peace

Romans 5:6

Christ arrives right on time to make this happen. He didn't, and doesn't, wait for us to get ready. (MSG)

Anxious
Because of
Cancer
Diagnosis - but
Even though I
Fear – I know
God
Has a plan

Instead of fear, I choose
Jesus to
Keep me at peace – to

Look at things positively – to
Make a conscious effort to avoid
Negativity – to
Open my heart to
Peace

Quiet time is essential

Rest imperative

Seeking God to
Teach me to
Understand His
Voice
Which
eXpands my heart
Yoking us together in His
Zone

November 4, 2021

I'm leaving you well and whole. That's my parting gift to you. Peace. I don't leave you the way you're used to being left—feeling abandoned, bereft. So don't be upset. Don't be distraught. (John 14:27, MSG)

May I pray for you and me?

Heavenly Father, we are happy you sent Jesus to become like one of us. We know You want us well, mentally, physically and spiritually. Yoke us to You so we can be in a strong connection with You. In Jesus' Name. Amen.

Journal Your Thoughts

Accepted

1 Peter 2:9-10

But you are God's chosen treasure—priests who are kings, a spiritual "nation" set apart as God's devoted ones. He called you out of darkness to experience his marvelous light, and now he claims you as his very own. He did this so that you would broadcast his glorious wonders throughout the world. For at one time you were not God's people, but now you are. At one time you knew nothing of God's mercy, because you hadn't received it yet, but now you are drenched with it. (TPT)

Accepted
Because
He cared for me - Jesus
Died
Even
For me

God opened
Heaven for me
Instilled in me hope
Just because He cared

Kept after me
Letting me question
Many times
Never turning aside

Opened my heart
Put everything right

Quite the accomplishment

Rescued
Solidifying our relationship

Total mercy
Unveiling the truth
Voicing His goals for me
Which I hope I am doing

eXcited to see where
Yonder is

Zealous for Him.

November 10, 2021

Cast all your anxiety on him because he cares for you. (2 Peter 5:7, NIV)

May I pray for you and me?

Heavenly Father, we are grateful to be one of the family. You adopted us. You claimed us. We are loved. Help us to hear Your goals for us. In Jesus' Name. Amen.

Journal Your Thoughts

My Dad, His Walk, the War

Journal Entry:

"Between the crosses, row on row," from the poem "In Flanders Fields" by John McCrae. That poem always stirs my thoughts to my Dad and how with God's help, he survived his time in WWII. My sister and I are grateful for our parents who instilled in us how to love one another, how to accept all peoples and how to be respectful to everyone.

This is a time of remembering. Remembering and having gratitude for our freedom.

I decided to reread my Dad's journal from D-Day. He landed First Wave on Juno Beach. What astounded me is the number of times he said, "It just missed us." Or "We were out of there before our position got bombed."

God is with us through all our trials. We are never alone. And for those whose lives we lost, we are forever grateful for their sacrifice. Lest we forget.

During this cancer journey, I have had such peace from all the prayers. And peace from God, Himself, as I read His Word faithfully every day and journal my thoughts.

I remember seeing my parents kneeling at their bedside together in prayer. I have an indelible picture of that in my head. My Dad knew he was saved for a purpose. He lived his life as an example of goodness, kindness, and respecting everyone. He was truly a gentle man of God.

There is something special about the poem when I read, "between the crosses." God is there in that field. He mourned over their losses. He knew the cost. His One and Only Son died on a cross.

I wrote a poem after reading my Dad's journal.

1 Peter 2:16-17

Live as free people, but do not use your freedom as a cover-up for evil; live as God's slaves. Show proper respect to everyone, love the family of believers, fear God, honor the emperor. (NIV)

Although my Dad didn't talk much about the War
Because he wanted to live in the present – he still
Created a record of
D-Day, the
Efforts, the
Frustrations, the
Guns

He kept all his feelings to himself and
Instead of burdening us he
Journaled
Kept notes, maps, pictures, uniforms, and helmets

Letting the past
Move back – it was
Necessary to
Open a new door

Putting his family first
Quieten his spirit
Rest in God
Seek to get along with others

Taught his children kindness
Understood to live his purpose, it was
Vital to live in the present

Walked daily with Jesus
eXcited to see the blessings as
Years flew by until his
Zed (February 15, 1993)

November 11, 2021

Rather, it should be that of your inner self, the unfading beauty of a gentle and quiet spirit, which is of great worth in God's sight. (1 Peter 3:4, NIV)

May I pray for you and me?

Heavenly Father, we thank You for teaching us to learn to get along with others. We thank You for teaching us to be humble of heart. We thank You for those who served to protect our freedoms. In Jesus' Name. Amen.

Journal Your Thoughts

Pray Continually

Journal Entry:

After all the comments to my cancer update (no cancer in sentinel nodes), I wrote this abecedarian poem today.

Ephesians 6:18

And pray in the Spirit on all occasions with all kinds of prayers and requests. With this in mind, be alert and always keep on praying for all the Lord's people. (NIV)

Absolutely
Blown away by
Caring friends

Didn't know that
Each person would pray

Finding that
God
Has built a team
Instructed them to pray

Jesus teaches us to
Keep praying
Love one another
Mention

Names
Often in our
Prayers

Questions answered

Resting in God's
Sustaining Presence as He
Teaches me
Underlying meanings of His Voice in His
Word

eXpanding my
Yearning to continue my
Zeal for Jesus

November 17th, 2021

Pray without ceasing. (1 Thessalonians 5:17, ESV)

Be constant in prayer. (Romans 12:12, ESV)

May I pray for you and me?

Heavenly Father, we long to hear Your voice. We know it takes practice. Continue to teach us how to pray. Help us learn to listen to Your voice. In Jesus' Name. Amen.

Journal Your Thoughts

God's Presence Scatters Fear

2 Corinthians 10:5

We demolish arguments and every pretension that sets itself up against the knowledge of God, and we take captive every thought to make it obedient to Christ. (NIV)

Anticipating the
Battle
Can cause
Distress

Evoking
Fear but
God brings
Hope
In
Jesus

Keeps all in perspective
Loves us fiercely

Makes
Nerves calm

Opens a way through
Prayer

Quashes
Ripples of
Severe
Terror that could overwhelm

Uses His Spirit to
Validate life

Wants to
X-irradiate
Your fear to
Zero

November 19, 2021

Do not be anxious about anything, but in every situation, by prayer and petition, with thanksgiving, present your requests to God. And the peace of God, which transcends all understanding, will guard your hearts and your minds in Christ Jesus. (Philippians 4:6-7, NIV)

May I pray for you and me?

Heavenly Father, speak into our hearts of Your peace. Help us not to fear. Calm our nerves. Help us hold tight to You, Jesus. Help us to take captive every thought that is not about You. In Your Name, we pray. Amen.

Journal Your Thoughts

After the Surgery

Journal Entry:

Sometimes I feel as if I am in a desert. We used to visit the desert of Arizona in the winter. And yes, I felt more thirsty there than I do here. At the moment, I am feeling parched. I need more of God.

Psalm 63

You, God, are my God,
earnestly I seek you;
I thirst for you,
my whole being longs for you,
in a dry and parched land
where there is no water. (NIV)

After
Breast
Cancer surgery

Don't
Expect
Full recovery immediately

God
Heals
Inside first

Jumping in too quickly
Keeps my body from finding a
Level that will
Make me heal

Note where pain strikes
Often not where I expect
Put a
Query to others

Rest and more rest
Supersedes
Tasks

Understand my body and mind
Variety is essential
Walking a daily routine

eXpect ups and downs

Yes, God surrounds me
Zealously

November 20, 2021

In peace I will lie down and sleep,
*   for you alone, Lord,*
*   make me dwell in safety. (Psalm 4:8, NIV)*

May I pray for you and me?

Heavenly Father, we come to You for our rest. We know we require it. Surround us with Your presence and peace. Heal us. In Jesus' Name. Amen.

Journal Your Thoughts

To the God Who Is Able

Now to him who is able to do immeasurably more than all we ask or imagine, according to his power that is at work within us. (Ephesians 3:20, NIV)

Am grateful
Because I know God
Can
Do this with little
Effort on my part

Focus on
God

Hesitate sometimes but
Instead refocus on
Jesus who
Keeps me calm and
Loving

Meditate on His Word
Notice new thoughts
Opens ideas
Puts things in perspective
Quickens my Spirit pushing

Restlessness aside
Silences the fearful
Thoughts

Unleashes a
Variety of
Words

eXpecting
Your
Zealousness for me

November 26, 2021

Rejoice always, pray continually, give thanks in all circumstances; for this is God's will for you in Christ Jesus. (1 Thessalonians 5:16-18, NIV)

May I pray for you and me?

Heavenly Father, we know from Your Word, that You are with us in all circumstances. We give You thanks for this life. We trust You to do more than we can ask or imagine. In Jesus' Name. Amen.

Journal Your Thoughts

End Zone

Matthew 11:28-30

Come to me, all you who are weary and burdened, and I will give you rest. Take my yoke upon you and learn from me, for I am gentle and humble in heart, and you will find rest for your souls. For my yoke is easy and my burden is light. (NIV)

Alpha
Before all
Christ existed

Death could not hold Him
Everlasting
Freedom for us

God in
Heaven
Invested in us

Jesus
Kept the Promise of God's
Love for us

Many will know
No stone unturned

Offers us
Peace in our hearts
Quiets our souls
Rest for the weary
Silence before the Lord

Toward the
Ultimate end
Victory over Satan

We're near the

eXit
Your end
Zone

December 12, 2021

For to us a child is born,
to us a son is given,
and the government will be on his shoulders.
And he will be called
Wonderful Counselor, Mighty God,
Everlasting Father, Prince of Peace. (Isaiah 9:6, NIV)

May I pray for you and me?

Heavenly Father, thank You for Jesus. We can learn from Him. We can give all our trials to Him. Jesus has conquered the grave. Therefore, we can live in peace knowing He has won the victory. In His Name, we pray. Amen.

Journal Your Thoughts

What's on My Mind?
COVID!!!

Journal Entry:

Two of my grandchildren have Covid. Both parents, vaccinated, are negative. Because I had some contact, I had to put radiation treatment on hold until I got my test which, praise God, is negative.

Both kids seem to have mild symptoms. I'm praying. I start radiation today, delayed from Monday.

Psalm 24:17

Wait for the Lord;
be strong and take heart
and wait for the Lord.

Another wait - this time
Because of
Covid

Dastardly plague
Entering our world
Finding victims

God - we cry out
Keep us safe

Love us
Make us more
Open to
Prayer

Quicken our hearts
Revive our
Spirits
Touch lives

Unleash Your
Voice to be heard
Willingly

eXcite
Your people with
Zeal

December 15, 2021

We wait in hope for the Lord;
    he is our help and our shield. (Psalm 33:20, NIV)

May I pray for you and me?

Heavenly Father, waiting is very hard. We are a people who want things right away. I am reminded of the Israelites in the desert. They couldn't wait for Moses to return and took things into their own hands. Help us to trust in You and wait for Your lead. As we continue to fight the battle with Covid, we ask for wisdom and patience. In Jesus' Name. Amen.

Journal Your Thoughts

ABCs of God

Isaiah 53:5

But he was pierced for our transgressions,
he was crushed for our iniquities;
the punishment that brought us peace was on him,
and by his wounds we are healed. (NIV)

Alpha
Blessed
Comforter
Defender
Eternal
Forever
God
Holy Spirit
Immanuel
Jesus
King
Living stone
Master
Name above all names
Omnipotent
Protector
Righteous One
Shepherd
Teacher

Unchangeable
Victorious
Wise
eXalted
Yesterday, today and forever
Zealous

December 17, 2021

Hear us, Shepherd of Israel,
you who lead Joseph like a flock;
You who sit enthroned between the cherubim,
shine forth. (Psalm 80:1, NIV)

May I pray for you and me?

Heavenly Father, there are so many names for You. They are all wonderful. Help us to study them all and know You more fully. Remind us that Jesus is our Shepherd, the Lion of Judah who knows us completely. In His Name, we pray. Amen.

Journal Your Thoughts

Get Dressed

Luke 11:33-36

You will be a shining lamp, reflecting rays of the truth by the way you live. (TPT)

Get up
Enter His Presence with
Thanks and praise

Don
Righteousness
Empathy
Sympathy

Stand strong in Christ

Enter the world
Dressed for His glory

January 12, 2022

Be kind and compassionate to one another, forgiving each other, just as in Christ God forgave you. (Ephesians 4:32, NIV)

May I pray for you and me?

Heavenly Father, in order to thrive in this world we need to stand strong in Christ. We need to work at being and acting as He did. We want to shine His light. Help us to do that. In Jesus' Name. Amen.

Journal Your Thoughts

Dig Deeper

Journal Entry:

I've decided to read a verse a week and memorize it. But I will also study it using the S.I.M.P.LE. Method of Bible study which I developed. I want to go deeper into God's Word. This time it's an alphabetical study.

Psalm 36:7

How priceless is your unfailing love, O God!
People take refuge in the shadow of your wings. (NIV)

Alphabetical study of God's Word
Becomes a place to
Concentrate, to
Dig deeper
Effectively.

Fresh ideas
God taught

Heaven appears
Inviting me in

Jesus opens the door
Kept closed by pride

Love flows
Multiplying each day

Never before has the door been so
Open

Peeking into Heaven
Quickening my heart
Rescuing my soul

Seek refuge under His wing
Time stands still
Understanding awakens

Veracity shown through the
Words of God
eXciting me

Yearning increases my
Zeal

January 15, 2022

All Scripture is God-breathed and is useful for teaching, rebuking, correcting and training in righteousness, so that the servant of God may be thoroughly equipped for every good work. (2 Timothy 3:16-17, NIV)

May I pray for you and me?

Heavenly Father, help us to desire to read Your Word on a regular basis. Help us to remember to pray before reading it. Help us catch fresh ideas and gather wisdom as we read Your Word. In Jesus' Name. Amen.

Journal Your Thoughts

Epilogue

As I start the work of publishing this book, I thought I would bring you up-to-date on my journey so far.

I've learned much about myself through this. My faith is stronger. I know who Jesus is and I will let my life be in His hands.

I've learned more about my body. I thought I had been eating well. Now I eat even more fruits, vegetables, nuts. I drink lots of water. My body needs to move. Exercise is very important. Although we have always walked 30 minutes a day, I sat too much. Now I get up from that position and move around. I have started core exercises to strengthen my back.

I continue to journal. Using my S.I.M.P.L.E. method of study helps me to go deeper into God's Word. I look at references, sit still and think about the passage, pray and listen to God. I have three published journals at the moment, and one is for those on this cancer adventure.

I will chat with you at any time. Email me at authorjaniscox@gmail.com. Join my online Bible study group.

One important thing to do is to get a regular mammogram! It saved my life.

Many blessings to you,

Janis

About Author

In 2001, Janis Cox said, "Yes," to Jesus. She confessed her sins and felt His acceptance and forgiveness. From that moment on, her life has been filled with lots of adventure, watching what He will do next and participating with Him.

Janis is happily married for over 50 years to a wonderful, patient, tolerant man. They have three beautiful, loving children and seven industrious and happy grandchildren. Their Maltipoo, Snowball, is their exuberant companion.

Janis has written and published over ten books so far. You can find all her books on Amazon and on her website at www.janiscox.com.

As an artist, a writer and publisher (under the name of Butterfly Beacons), God is moving her step-by-step on the path He has laid out for her.

If you are looking for a safe place to study the Bible, join us in my private Facebook group: *Growing through God's Word*

Instagram: https://www.instagram.com/janis_cox

Twitter: https://twitter.com/AuthorJanisCox

LinkedIn: https://www.linkedin.com/in/authorjaniscox

Facebook (page): https://www.facebook.com/authorjaniscox

Janis has published another book about cancer: *S.I.M.P.L.E. Journal: Be a Cancer Thriver*